The Ultimate Guide to Sleep:
How to Combat Insomnia and Sleep Problems

Jessica Lopez

Table of Contents

Introduction

Having difficulties when it comes to sleeping? Do you find yourself wide-awake even though the clock ticks 1 in the morning? You may have Insomnia! Studies show that Insomnia or sleep disorder is affecting millions of individuals worldwide, and they have to live with this type of medical condition. These people find it difficult to stay asleep or fall asleep. Insomnia commonly leads to lethargy and sleepiness during daytime. There are even instances when the affected person would fee unwell both physically and mentally.

This book includes some general information about Insomnia; who gets it, what causes it, general signs and symptoms, the manner by which Insomnia is diagnosed and available treatment alternatives.

Thanks again for downloading this book, I hope it helps you combat Insomnia and Sleep Problems.

Join our Mailing List Today to Receive FREE Book Giveaways and Special Offers!

Chapter 1 - What is Insomnia?

Insomnia may include an extensive range of sleeping problems, from lack of quantity of sleep to absence of quality of sleep. Sleeplessness is commonly categorized into three types:

Chronic Insomnia – this kind would last for months, sometimes years. The national institute of health made a study, which shows that majority of chronic Insomnia instances, is considered secondary. This means that Insomnia is merely a symptom or a side effect of another problem.

Acute Insomnia – also referred to as short term Insomnia. The symptoms may persist for a number of weeks.

Transient Insomnia – this type of Insomnia occurs whenever symptoms last from several days to weeks.

Although Insomnia can affect individuals at any age, it's more common in adult women than adult men. The worst thing about this sleeping disorder is that it can undermine both work and school performance. It's also one of the most common causes of reduced reaction time, poor immune system function, concentration problems, irritability, depression, anxiety, and obesity. Insomnia has been associated with higher risks of developing chronic illnesses.

The National Sleep Foundation found out that between 30 percent and 40 percent of American adults have Insomnia symptoms within the past 12 months. Additionally, approximately 10 to 15 percent of adults claim to develop chronic Insomnia.

What are the Symptoms of Insomnia?

Insomnia isn't just about having a hard time sleeping. Even if you go to sleep exactly on 10PM every night, you might still suffer from the condition if you exhibit the following symptoms:

- Waking up in the middle of the night and having a hard time sleeping again

- Waking up several times throughout the night, usually around 3 to 5 times

- Necessitating sleeping pills to fall asleep on a regular basis

- Fragmented sleep and waking up utterly exhausted in the morning

- Continuous light sleeping during the night, causing you to feel tired by day

What Causes Insomnia?

The causes of Insomnia can be classified into physical and psychological factors. There's often a core medical condition, which causes chronic Insomnia. On the other hand, transient Insomnia may be caused by a recent occurrence or event.

Medications - according to AARP, an association of retired individuals in America, the following types of medications or drugs may cause Insomnia in some patients:

1. Statins – drugs used for curing high cholesterol level. Examples of this medication include: atorvastatin, lovastatin, rosuvastatin, and simvastatin.

2. Corticosteroids – drugs used for treating individuals with inflammation of the blood vessels and muscles, rheumatoid arthritis, lupus, gout, allergic reactions, and Sjögren's syndrome. Examples are: cortisone, methylprednisolone, triamcinolone, and prednisone.

3. Alpha blockers – this form of medication are commonly utilized for curing hypertension, benign prostatic hyperplasia or BPH, Raynaud's disease and high blood pressure. Examples are: tamsulosin, doxazosin, prazosin, alfuzosin, terazosin, and silodosin.

4. Beta blockers – they are used for treating irregular heartbeat or arrhythmias and hypertension. Examples are: sotalol, atenolol, prograpnolol, carvedilol and timolol.

5. SSRI antidepressants – drugs used for curing depression. Examples are: fluvoxamine, sertraline, escitalopram, paroxetine, citalopram and fluoxetine.

ACE inhibitors, Angiotensin II receptor blockers or ARBs, cholinesterase inhibitors, glucosamine or chondroitin, second generation or non-sedating H1 agonists may also cause sleeplessness.

Disruptions in one's circadian rhythm that is caused by hotness or coldness, noisiness, high altitudes, and job shift changes can also cause Insomnia. Psychological problems such as mood disorders, depression or bipolar disorder, anxiety, and psychotic disorders are more likely to cause Insomnia.

Certain medical conditions such as the following may also cause Insomnia: arthritis, Parkinson's sleep apnea, asthma, chronic obstructive pulmonary disease, acid reflux disease, angina, congestive heart failure, chronic fatigue, chronic pain, stroke, tumors and brain lesions. Other factors include any of the following: pregnancy, overactive mind, genetic conditions, parasites, or sleeping next to an individual who snores a lot.

When Should You Consult a Doctor?

Through the help of this book, you should be able to address insomnia yourself. If the condition is severely affecting the quality of your life, professional help might become necessary. Try out the self-help methods offered here and if none of them work, it is greatly encouraged that you consult a doctor. If you find yourself falling asleep during the day, even while performing activities, professional intervention is imminent.

Chapter 2 - Should you have Media Technology Inside your Room?

Media technology inside the bedroom can definitely disrupt one's sleep patterns especially that of children. Studies show that kids with video games, televisions, computers, mobile phones and DVD players in their bedrooms slept less than kids with no devices inside their rooms.

Who can be affected by Insomnia?

Some people are likely to suffer Insomnia compared to other people:

1. Menopausal women

2. Elderly

3. Shift workers with constant changes in shifts

4. Travelers

5. Adolescents or young adult students

6. Drug users

7. Those with mental disorders

How will Insomnia be cured?

Some kinds of Insomnia can be resolved whenever the underlying causes wear off or are removed. Generally, curing Insomnia concentrates on determining the root cause of the sleeping problem. Once identified, the underlying cause can be corrected or treated. In addition to curing the underlying reason or cause of Insomnia, both non-pharmacological and medical treatments may be utilized as adjuvant therapies.

Chapter 3 - Non-pharmacological Techniques in Curing Insomnia

Improve your "sleep time" – do not over or under sleep, get regular exercise, do not force yourself to sleep, always maintain your regular sleep schedule, do not drink coffee at night, don't smoke, don't go to bed with an empty stomach, make sure your environment is comfortable.

Make use of the right relaxation techniques – muscle relaxation and meditation.

Cognitive therapy – it can be in the form of group therapy or one-on-one type of counseling sessions.

Stimulus control therapy – make it a point to go to bed when you're already sleepy, avoid a long daytime nap, refrain from reading, watching TV, eating or getting anxious in bed, and set your clock to a daily alarm schedule.

Sleep restriction – if necessary, you need to decrease the amount of time you spend in bed. As much as possible, deprive your body of sleep. This way, you're more tired the following night.

Light Therapy – light is a very important aspect of sleeping within the right times. Light Therapy basically makes good use of this by exposing an insomniac to very specific light spectrums during the day and at nighttime. This helps the body efficiently distinguish between "night" and "day", therefore triggering melatonin production and easing the way to sleep. Light Therapy can be done by professionals although there are also products out in the market today in aid of this system. Light therapy lamps are currently available in many online stores.

Sleep Clinic – at some point, doctors may refer you to a sleep clinic where your brain patterns will be recorded during sleep. Medical professionals will then log in their findings and provide you with ideal treatments based on the results of the test. This is mostly done for chronic insomniacs who have tried all other options.

Sleep Diary – much like with a Food Diary, a Sleep Diary can offer you excellent insight on your sleeping habits and exactly what aspects might be causing your problem. The diary should include:

- Time you went to bed

- Estimated time that you went to sleep

- Intended time for waking up

- Actual time you woke up

- Feeling throughout the day (drowsy, energetic)

- How you woke up (using alarm clock or naturally)

- Exercises and preparation done before sleeping (meditation, stretches, etc)

- Type of sleep (fragmented, deep)

- Any dreams throughout the night

- Any pills/medication/food you took before going to sleep

- The number of times you woke up during the night and how long before you slept again

All these information can help you notice patterns with your sleeping condition. For example, you might notice that eating a burger before going to bed makes it harder for you to sleep. Being fully aware of these details can make it easier for you to eliminate or promote the factors that help/prevent you from experiencing a deep and satisfying sleep.

Common Medical Treatments for Insomnia

1. Antidepressants

2. Prescription sleeping pills such as benzodiazepines

3. Antihistamines

4. Over-the-counter sleep aids

5. Valerian officinalis

6. Ramelteon

7. Melatonin

Guidelines for Taking Pills for Insomnia

Although many anti-insomnia cures are available over the counter, it's crucial that you first assess your condition before purchasing one. Infrequent bouts of insomnia may be addressed with sleeping pills but if you're suffering from the condition for more than a week, a more direct approach might be necessary. Always follow the instructions provided in the medication labels.

For best results, only take sleeping pills if you still have enough time to sleep for the complete 8 hours. For example, taking one at 1AM will only leave you feeling exhausted and sleepy when you eventually wake up. Take the pills only when you're ready to sleep and keep in mind that alcohol and sleeping pills should NEVER be mixed.

In this 24/7 society, too many people see sleep as merely a luxury rather than an essential thing to do. Needless to say, there's no problem when it comes to spending long hours working and then adding several activities that can change a busy day into an optimistically grinding experience. Many workers delay their physical and mental recharge as they skimp on sleep. However, when they finally go to bed, their minds are restless and unwilling to rest.

Insomnia is a complex physical condition that is often caused by several factors. Addressing those factors frequently requires environment and lifestyle changes. When Insomnia strikes, an option is to choose prescription sleep aids. However, you have to remember that there are numerous effective natural sleep remedies that are currently made available to you. Changes in one's lifestyle, as well as herbal supplements, synthetic supplements, and food items may help you, consider trying several techniques to obtain a restful sleep.

Chapter 4 - Foods Herbs and Supplements: Best Natural Insomnia Remedies

Melatonin. This is a special type of hormone that can help in regulating a person's sleep and wake cycle. Experts are considering melatonin as an internal pacemaker that can regulate the timing and the drive for sleep in human beings. Further, it can also cause drowsiness, slow metabolic functions, lower body temperature, and put the body into the so-called "sleep mode".

Researches on melatonin in patients with Insomnia are mixed. A study shows that taking melatonin could improve and restore sleep in individuals with Insomnia. On the other hand, some studies illustrate that melatonin doesn't help patients with Insomnia stay asleep. It's also a fact that melatonin isn't regulated by the Food and Drugs Authority, and this can cause problems with purity.

It's only advised for individuals with circadian rhythm problems, and it should not be given to kids or taken by those who are still taking other forms of medications. It's important that you use melatonin only under close supervision by a physician.

Warm Milk. Why not put some spin on your grandmother's herbal Insomnia remedy? This can be done by sipping warm milk prior to bed. You have to drink something that has an excellent source of calcium like almond milk. This drink will help your brain to generate melatonin. Additionally, warm milk will spark pleasant as well as relaxing memories of your childhood. Think of the times when your mother was helping you fall asleep.

Snacks that will help you fall asleep. The best sleep-inducing food items include a perfect combination of carbohydrates and protein. A light snack which is composed of half a banana together with a whole-wheat cracker and cheese or one tablespoon of peanut butter will do. Consume one of these snacks 30 minutes before you hit the hay.

Magnesium. This item apparently plays an important role when it comes to the regulation of sleep. Studies show that even a marginal deficiency in magnesium can prevent one's brain from finally settling down at night. It's also true that an absorbable form of magnesium is the magnesium citrate powder that is available in several health food stores.

Why don't you try taking 2 doses a day? Just make sure to follow the direction label correctly. The second dose has to be taken before bedtime. You can also acquire magnesium from food. Excellent sources include almonds, pumpkin seeds, wheat germ, and green leafy vegetables.

Lavender. The soothing effect of lavender oil is already proven to provide the best relaxing effect. Lavender oil can help in calming one's mind; thereby, encouraging sleep in some individuals with Insomnia. Try taking a hot bath and place several drops of lavender oil. It will help relax your mind and body.

Valerian root. This special medicinal herb has been utilized to treat sleep issues since the time of the ancient civilization in Greece and Rome. Valerian root can be sedating and it can also help you fall asleep faster. Researches on the effective impact of valerian root for Insomnia are mixed. Some experts are saying that if the patient tries valerian as a sleep treatment, patience is required. It can several few hours for its sedating impact to take effect. It's important that you consult a doctor before you take valerian and don't forget to follow the label directions.

L-theanine. This is an amino acid that can be found on green tea. The main objective of using this item is to help combat anxiety since this type of mental condition certainly interferes with sleep. Recent studies showed that L-theanine could effectively reduce heart rate and immune response to stress. L-theanine can work by increasing the production of serotonin, the so-called feel-good hormone. It can also induce the brain waves that have great impact when it comes to relaxation. Before you take L-Theanine, it's important that you talk to your physician about any possible drug interactions.

Cherries. Cherries naturally contain melatonin, a popular factor that helps the body settle down for sleep. There are currently melatonin capsules being offered on the market – but why consume this if you have a natural option? Try eating a few fresh cherries or even drinking cherry juice before going to sleep. In small amounts taken overtime, you'll find that sleeping becomes easier. The fruit has been documented to work for chronic insomniacs as well.

Cereals. Cereals are great for breakfast but even better for dinner. It's filling enough to stave off hunger but light enough that you won't feel discomfort in the stomach. Opt for wheat-based cereal that contains complex carbohydrates perfect for the body. You can eat it as is or include some milk in the mix. What's great about this is that milk is also known for aiding sleep, letting you fully relax and drift off with no problem.

Of course, there are also some food items that you should AVOID to prevent insomnia. If some of these food types are in your daily diet, then don't be confused if you're having a hard time sleeping every night:

Cheeseburger. This fatty food, along with every other one with high-fat content, can be problematic when trying to go to sleep. The fat is basically hard to digest for the stomach, causing the acid to rise up and eventually lead to heartburn. The discomfort can make it hard for you to find a sleep-worthy position. If you have to, consume a burger hours before bedtime to empty your stomach of the fat content.

Coffee. This one's pretty obvious but a lot of people do it anyway. Keep in mind that coffee contains caffeine which boosts the body's nervous system, essentially "waking" us up. Coffee – even a decaffeinated one – should be limited to daytime use.

Dark Chocolate. Dark chocolate is basically like coffee when it comes to caffeine content. Not to mention all the calories that comes with each bite. To play it safe, avoid all types of chocolate being going to bed.

Alcohol. Some people use alcohol to "wind down" after a long day and help them go to sleep. Although this is often effective, alcohol can create a dependency that you don't want. Drinking more than one glass can also change the results completely, leaving you awake half the night. Should you be able to sleep, waking up several times through the night is possible.

Please note that different food items affect people differently. A sleep diary would be able to help you track what food items help or trigger your insomnia. There are also instances when specific food types not only cause insomnia but also lead to nightmares when a person eventually falls asleep. All of these should be recorded in your sleep diary for future reference.

Chapter 5 - Natural Sleep Remedies: Change your Lifestyle

The following modifications to your lifestyle as well as the environment can help combat sleep issues:

Switch the television off.

In some individuals, nighttime light may inhibit melatonin, and this will further create "social jetlag". This type of condition would mimic several symptoms of having taken a trip to several time zones. In order to make sure that your bedroom is as dark as possible, it is recommended that you move the television out of your bedroom. You may simply use a TIVO or a DVR to record your favorite late night show for your later viewing.

Other gadgets should be placed away from the bed.

For those who really want a good and restful sleep, it's important that you turn your appliances away. Take them out of your bed. Or better yet, you could turn them off altogether. In addition, if you must utilized bedroom electronics, choose those items with illuminated red light. Red light is less disturbing when it comes to melanin production, so it's a lot better compared to blue light.

If you're still awake after thirty minutes, give it up.

If you do not fall asleep within a period of thirty minutes, sleep experts recommend that you get up, leave your room and read. Perform some exercise or do whatever it is that can help tire you out. Meditation is also a good way to spend time before getting to bed. When you feel tired again, you may return to bed.

Keep the pets separated.

If you allow your pets to sleep in your room, chances are they might be the reason for your sleep problems. Dogs and cats can become active during night time, often waking up and consequently waking you up from slumber. If this happens often, it might be best to train your dog/cat into sleeping in his own corner of the house.

Music.

White noise is not the only thing you can use to help you fall asleep. A soothing song or even a meditation script can lead you to a drowsy relaxed state. Find the audio that makes you feel utterly content and listen to it before going to bed. Better yet, create a playlist that you can start playing every time, allowing your body's tension and energy to deplete and eventually lead you to sleep.

Massage.

Try asking your significant other for a relaxing massage before going to sleep. You can also hire people for the job although keep in mind that this can be expensive. If a massage is not possible, you can also try soaking in a hot and relaxing bath, preferably with some flowery scents added to the mix. Heat actually helps release tension in the muscles, making it easier for you to curl up and go to sleep.

Enjoy the sun.

The sun has incredible sleep-related powers that artificial light can never replicate. If you spend your days in the office, it's strongly advised that you stand under the sun and let the warmth soothe your skin. Do these for at least one hour each day, making sure that you get the "early" rays when the heat isn't too painful on the skin. This gives your body an excellent point of reference when establishing an internal clock.

Meditation for insomnia

Meditation has been proven as one of the most effective ways to go to sleep. Studies suggest that insomniacs who practice meditation fall asleep in half the time they normally do. To perform meditation conducive for sleep, try assuming a lying down pose. Keep your body relaxed and start concentrating on your breathing. Try to visualize a flower the opens when you take in a breath and expands as your expel air. Become more aware of your surroundings, feeling how hot/cold the temperature is and the bed sheets as it rests on your skin. Although instant sleep is not possible on your first try, repeated attempts can help with insomnia. Meditation primarily works because it lets you concentrate on other things other than the fact that you're not asleep. Through a misdirected focus, the brain activity slows down and you'll stop worrying about the events of the day or what will happen tomorrow.

Early workouts work for some people.

It's no secret that workouts promote a restful sleep as well as a good overall health. But, a study that has been published in the journal showed that the type of workout and the specific time of day when it's done certainly make a difference. Additionally, researchers found that females who exercised within a moderate intensity for 30 minutes every morning, 7 days a week, are having less trouble when it comes to sleeping than females who work out less or later during the day. Morning workouts seem to affect the rhythm of the body which would later affect one's quality of sleep.

Enjoy sex

Sex is one of the most enjoyable ways to fall asleep. It manages to accomplish two things: give you a good workout and help the muscles feel relaxed and lethargic. Take advantage of your insomniac state and have a little fun with your significant other. An active bout of sex can leave you sleepy in a matter of minutes.

Wind down.

Just because you're in your pajama doesn't mean you'd fall asleep as soon as your head hits the pillow. You can't just turn "on" and "off" with sleep and instead, you'll need to ease your way into bedtime. This means going through a relaxing routine that gives your body time to de-stress. This can be something as simple as taking a hot shower, brushing your teeth and wearing your pajamas. If you have a beauty routine then this would also suffice, as long as the steps do not trigger your body to start pumping adrenaline. If you repeat these steps every night, the body starts to develop a pattern and recognize that it's time to "shut down".

One of the reasons why this type of interplay between sleep and exercise exists may be the person's body temperature. The temperature rises during workouts and takes up to six hours for it to drop down to normal. Cooler body temperatures are commonly associated with a much better sleep; hence, it's important that you give your body enough time to cool off prior to sleeping.

Your slumber surroundings should always be kept tranquil.

The bedroom has to feel like a sanctuary for you. It follows that piles of clothes that are thrown on the bed, stacks of bills, as well as other clutter will only hamper you emotionally; thereby, leading to sleep problems. An organized and tranquil space will make you feel relaxed. So, to create a perfect sleep environment for you, try the following:

You may wear your pajamas to bed. This will signal your mind that it's finally bedtime.

Your room should be kept cool, between 65 to 72 degrees. This is the optimal range of temperature for sleeping.

Try making your room darker. Consider installing the right shades that will make your room appear dark. Or better yet, wear eye covers that can block the light from the LED displays or the streets.

Spray your favorite smell around the room – something soothing and helps you get in that "peaceful" place, perfect for sleep.

Purchase a good mattress. Remember that you're spending one-third of your life in bed. Don't you think purchasing a good mattress is a good investment?

Use a pillow that can support your neck and head. Give your pillow a bend test; it should not be too floppy such that if you're going to bend the pillow in half, it should stay in position.

You could make use of a white noise machine in order to filter the unwanted sound. The brain would still hear things whenever you sleep.

Make sure that you're using breathable linens. These items will reduce skin irritation, body odor, and sweat – all of which can disrupt your rest or sleep.

Natural sleep therapy can do wonders for infrequent bouts of poor sleep. But, they should not be utilized for chronic sleep issues. If you are experiencing Insomnia, which lasts for several weeks or even more, it's important that you consult your physician.

How to Sleep

Are you having trouble getting to bed? Well, you are not alone! The NSF or national sleep foundation illustrates that more than fifteen percent of American adults are having issues in sleeping. There are a few things, which are more significant to one's overall health than having a good sleep. It's a good thing that a good night's sleep may be several short steps away. Start curing your Insomnia by enhancing your room's design. This way, you can attain maximum tranquility.

Select the Most Suitable Color

The type of paint for your bedroom walls as well as the colors you utilize to decorate can certainly affect the way you think and feel while you are inside your bedroom. Ultimately, this can affect your sleep. Researches have shown that subdued colors of green and blue can elicit right feelings such as calmness, comfort, relaxation, hope and peace. Lighter shades such as tan and peach may also help in calming your senses prior to bedtime.

You have to get the Right Bed

Since you spend one third of your time in bed, it would make sense for you to commit some time and money in purchasing the most suitable bed. There's no such thing as a one-size-fits-all type of mattress. You have to find a store that will let you test the mattress for at least thirty days prior to buying the same. Try various types of pillows and choose the right size and level of firmness that a good mattress should have. If you usually wake up sore or stiff, you should try something else.

Turning Down the Lights

Your body has to be conditioned that it's already time to sleep. Hence, it would greatly help if you turn down the lights. It seems obvious, but make certain that the room is dark enough in order for your body to fall asleep faster. It's also a must that you turn off every light source. Close the curtain or blinds. Remember that even moonlight streetlights can disrupt your sleep. For those who need some light in order to fall asleep, you may get a nightlight. This dim or switch-controlled lamp will emit dim light so your sleep will not be disrupted.

Turn the Clock

Turn your alarm clock. It should be facing away from the bed. Experts say that this is the simplest, but most effective type of adjustment. Low light that comes from the clock can even affect your sleep. You will only be watching the clock ticking as you lie flat in bed. If this is the case, you'll be suffering from mental stress which may prevent you from relaxing and sleeping.

Don't place a television set or a computer inside your bedroom.

Even though you may be tempted to simply curl up and start watching a movie while staying comfortable in bed, always remember that your bedroom should only be confined or reserved for intimacy and sleeping. Electronics or gadgets can affect your sleep. Move your TV set into another room.

However, if you're using your bedroom as a mini-office, or home office, make certain that the moment you put away your personal computer, it's already out of sight. Also, you have to be sure that there is no soft blue glow or light that's coming from your cellular phone, iPod, Kindle or either.

Organize or De-clutter

Organize the shelves and closet so that there will be no piles of clothes as well as stacks of books that will be lying around the room. Start moving unfinished projects or works out of the bedroom so they will never stress you out whenever you are getting ready to sleep. Uncluttered rooms will result to an uncluttered mind, easy relaxation and less distraction.

The air inside your home and bedroom should be clean.

You will have a quality sleep when you can breathe easier. Open the windows often to allow fresh air to enter your bedroom. You may want to install air-purifying plants or a filter or air-purifying system to rid the air inside the room of allergens and toxins. Finally, consider aromatherapy. Start sprinkling mist in your pillow, and this can be done by infusing water with vanilla, lavender, bergamot, sandalwood or chamomile. The scent coming from these items will soothe your senses.

Still Can't Sleep?

After you have redesigned your bedroom and did everything to ensure that the lights are out, but still lie awake at night, this may be the right time for you to take further steps. Make use of several small behavioral modifications that can be made during day time. This will certainly pay huge dividends during sleep time. You may consider this extensive list of Insomnia remedies. You should never accept a life without sleep. Certainly, you deserve better!

Chapter 6 - Home Remedies for Insomnia

It's 5 in the morning, and the first trace of dawn begun to come out in the nighttime sky. You have been awake since 2 in the morning, and are starting to feel hopeless. Your major concern is how you'll be able to function or work well? You still have a presentation to accomplish and your mind isn't focused yet. So, will you be capable of going through another day without sleep?

Physicians say that adults require an average of 7 to 9 hours of sleep every night, but Insomnia can certainly keep them from sleeping right. One of the most common sleep problems in Europe and North America is Insomnia. One-third of the entire United States population can't sleep well; thus, cannot function well during daytime. Half of those individuals have 1 or 2 bad nights per week, and the other half would spend countless sleepless nights turning, tossing and feeling miserable. These people likewise spend countless days of being exhausted.

The following remedies will help ease the symptoms of Insomnia:

1. Make sure that you sleep in a quiet room. If you can hear even a slight sound, you have to wear earplugs. Remember that the most excellent sleep environment should be one that's cool, comfortable, quiet and dark.

2. Your pillow should not be too soft or too hard.

3. Limit your alcohol and caffeine consumption. Even though alcohol can make you drowsy and sleepy, it has an unpleasant adverse effect – it can wake you up later at night with a full bladder, stomachache or a headache. On the other hand, caffeine can stimulate your brain. You have to limit the coffee intake to 2 cups daily.

4. Keep a regular schedule. One of the most important rules for individuals with Insomnia is to maintain a normal sleep schedule. If you cannot sleep one night, then get up the next morning at your usual time, and avoid taking any naps.

5. Learn to establish your bed time ritual. A hot bath taken 2 hours before bedtime would be good as it can stimulate sleep. Of course, there may be several exceptions so you have to experiment on the right timing. Other people believe that bathing will delay bedtime; for some, it's the other way around.

6. Naturopathic practitioners suggest adding 1 to 2 cups of Epsom salt to their hot bath. They soak their body for 15 to 20 minutes prior to hitting the hay.

7. You could try a little sugar. Finish eating 2 to 3 hours prior to bedtime. Sugary foods consumed about thirty minutes prior to bedtime can act as a sedative. You can wake up with no morning fuzziness which accompanies synthetic sleeping pills.

8. Honey has a similar sedative impact as sugar. It may allow you to sleep quickly. You should try adding one tablespoon of honey to a decaffeinated herbal tea or warm milk to obtain that relaxing, pre-sleep drink.

9. Don't you love to take a snack, but how about taking it before bedtime? A high carbohydrate and low protein bedtime snack can make you feel sleepy. Carbohydrate-rich food items such as toast tend to produce the right effect on the tummy. It can also ease the brain and create that blissful slumber.

10. Of course, who would ever forget drinking one glass of warm milk prior to bedtime? It's already an age-old cure for sleeping problems. Several scientists believe that the presence of the chemical tryptophan plays an important role. It can help the brain ease up into a sleep mode. Milk seems to help individuals hit the sack easily. It can effectively relax the body and the mind. But, if you frequently wake up to urinate, it's important that you avoid liquids several hours prior to bedtime.

Other food items that are high on tryptophan are the following: tuna, soybeans, turkey, chicken, cashews, and cottage cheese.

Experts likewise believe that deficiency in tryptophan can cause issues with sleep. Items such as sleep supplements can help the body create serotonin. Low serotonin levels are one of the known factors that cause sleepless nights. Sleep supplements may benefit your body by causing the mind to relax a bit. A low level of tryptophan is common in individuals who are experiencing depression. If your Insomnia problems are connected with depression, it's important that you ask your doctor.

Chapter 7 – Other Sleep Disorders

Insomnia is the most popular sleep disorder – but it's not the only one. There are also other sleeping problems that you might misdiagnose as "insomnia". Here's a list of common sleep disorders and their accompanying symptoms.

Delayed Sleep Phase

Delayed Sleep Phase is when your body recognizes a skewed 24-hour body clock. For example, you tend to feel sleepy around 2AM and wake up around 10AM. Although you still get your 8-hour's worth of sleep, you're getting them at incorrect times of the day. In most cases, this leads you to feel groggy after waking up, feeling as though you're incredibly exhausted even though you just woke up.

It's interesting to note that DSP is often misdiagnosed as insomnia, therefore resulting to a misdirected treatment. Study reveals that the condition requires a very different approach which may include pharmacologic and non-pharmacologic options. Light therapy, intake of melatonin,

Shift Working Disorder

This type of sleep disorder is very common in the modern world where some jobs have changing shifts. Doctors, nurses, firemen and other careers necessitating 24-hour presence often suffer most from this condition. Basically, people with a Shift Working Sleep Disorder have changing sleep patterns, causing confusion to their bodies. They might be on duty at night for one week and then expected to work daytime for the second week. Fortunately, there are ways to handle this type of problem without having to change your job:

Consciously use more light when you're working to fool the body – especially if you're on the night shift. On the other hand, make sure that there is zero light when you're about to go to sleep. If your sleeping time happens to be in the middle of the day, it's best to dim your room as much as possible. Use heavy drapes, close the windows or cover your eyes to prevent light from pouring in.

Avoid using electronics hours before sleeping. This should help speed up your body's adjustment and therefore make it easier for you to sleep.

Minimize shift changes as much as possible. If you can, request shift changes that are later rather than earlier. The body find it easier to adjust to later sleeping time rather than earlier ones.

Restless Leg Syndrome

Restless Leg Syndrome abbreviated to RLS is also misdiagnosed as insomnia. As the name suggests, the condition is characterized by the need to move your arms or legs when lying down. The constant movement therefore prevents you from falling asleep, hence the mistaken belief that it is actually insomnia. RLS is concentrated on these two body parts and usually happens because the sufferer feels a strange sensation in the legs/arms. Constant leg jerking and cramping might also be evident. The tingling or aching in the legs disappear each time you move, massage or stretch the legs.

There are some common treatments between Restless Leg Syndrome and insomnia. Some of the natural techniques you can try out include:

- Moderate leg stretches and exercises

- Massaging the legs

- Soaking in the bathtub to fully relax yourself

- Going to sleep at the same time each day

- Weight loss

- Avoiding alcohol, caffeine and cigarettes

Jet Lag

Jet lag is a phenomenon when the body's circadian rhythm is interrupted due to changing time zones. If you're a frequent flyer then chances are you suffer from this condition often. According to studies, the technique to dealing with jet lag is to acclimatize yourself to the new time zone. For example, if you leave in time for dinner and arrive in time for lunch, it's important to delay sleep until its bedtime for your new time zone. Doing so helps your internal clock adjust to the new "time", allowing you to feel sleepy, experience hunger or feel energized at the correct times.

If you know you're travelling between two different time zones, it's best to start adjusting your body clock in preparation. For example, if you're going somewhere a few hours advance to your current time zone, try going to sleep one hour before your usual bedtime. You can also try waking up an hour ahead of your usual waking hours until your body gets used to the system. By the time you fly out, there shouldn't be any "jet lag" problems in your new location.

Narcolepsy

Narcolepsy is a more serious form of sleep disorder that affects the brain patterns. The most obvious characteristic of the condition is when a person experiences extreme drowsiness in the daytime, causing them to fall asleep. In some cases, the need to sleep overtakes them even if they're doing something that requires focus such as eating, driving, exercising, cooking and others. Other symptoms of the condition include having dreams the instant you fall asleep and inability to move when you're about to wake up. Narcolepsy is typically treated by professional, referring patients to a support group and adequate lifestyle changes.

Sleep Apnea

This is a serious form of sleep disorder, often life threatening for its sufferers. The condition is characterized by suddenly stopping mid-breath during sleep. The chances of developing the condition include being overweight, a smoker or someone who has a relative suffering from the same problem. Note that sleep apnea may be misdiagnosed as insomnia because the sufferers often feel sleepy and lethargic in the morning. They also suffer from interrupted sleeps throughout the night, often waking up every few hours. Sleep apnea requires a very different set of treatments compared to insomnia.

If you're in doubt about what sleeping disorder you're suffering from, consulting a professional is usually best. Keep in mind that not all these sleeping disorders can be addressed at home so self-diagnosis and treatment would not really work.

Chapter 8 – Ultimate Insomnia Cure and FAQ

If your insomnia is getting out of control and already affecting your quality of life, a more severe action may be necessary. According to psychologist, the ultimate insomnia cure is camping. The information was published in 2013 in the *Current Biology* journal, revealing that the participants experienced synchronization in their sleeping habits in just one week of camping. The results were even the same whether the participant is a self-confessed night owl or early riser.

The Circadian Rhythm is basically a person's internal clock. This is triggered by the light turning on and turning off. In the old days when there's no artificial light, the rhythm is dependent on the rising and setting of the sun. When sunlight comes pouring in, the body is "switched on" and a person wakes up. As the sun sets, the body goes to sleep in order to regain lost energy.

Camping outside basically helps reboot a person's Circadian Rhythm, allowing it to get back on track. See, modern technology especially artificial lighting tends to "fool" the body's internal clock. For millions of years, the sun has been used by the body as a signal of when to "wake up" and "shut down". Unfortunately, it's hard for the body to distinguish between fluorescent lighting and the illumination from the sun, therefore causing confusion and eventually, insomnia. In one week of relying only on sunlight however, a person's Circadian Rhythm can be "rebooted", allowing him/her to get back to healthy sleeping hours.

When camping outdoors to treat insomnia, following are some important things to keep in mind:

There should be zero artificial lighting anywhere. This means leaving behind your laptop and mobile phones and get really in touch with nature. If leaving your phone is not possible, make sure that it is only used when necessary or when the sun is up. Even a flashlight is not advisable.

The only allowable light during camping is a campfire. Studies reveal that even the color of the light deeply affects insomnia in many patients. However, the natural color of fire will not affect a person's sleeping problems.

In the morning, try to absorb as much light as possible to boost your body's energy. Go fishing, hiking or trekking, making sure that your body fully adjusts to the light of the sun. Of course, don't forget to protect yourself using a hat and some sunscreen, just in case.

At night, allow yourself to enjoy the sunset and soak in the stars. The changing colors of the sky can unconsciously trigger the body in readiness for sleep. The sunset is also known for relaxing individuals, both in mind and spirit.

Don't forget to still follow a strict bedtime during camping. Around 10PM would be great since this offers you sufficient time to grab your 8 hours of sleep. Just remember – you are basically resetting your body clock at this point. When you go home, you would likely need to sleep at the same time as when you do during camping.

It's important to note that one week camping doesn't just cure insomnia but also other sleep-related problems such as fragmented sleep, jet lag, an shift working disorder. If you tend to wake up in the middle of the night or wake up still feeling tired, camping can offer a solution. Of course, some sleeping disorders such as sleep apnea cannot be easily addressed through simple camping as they have very different trigger. Note though that one week of sunlight-only exposure is the minimum recommended length of time. Any less than that and you might not get the results you want.

Of course, not everyone might have the time or inclination to go camping. Fortunately, it's possible to try this out without leaving home. Simply make sure that NO artificial lighting is switched on at night and make good use of candles for illumination. Pretend that there's a mass power shortage every time the sun starts to set. Make sure the candle is no longer burning before going to bed and do NOT use mobile phones/computers when the light from the sun is gone.

I have a heart condition. Is it OK to take sleeping pills?

If you have health problems, it's always best to consult your doctor before taking sleeping pills, even if they're over the counter medication. The reason for this is that the introduction of new chemicals can aggravate your problem. If you're already taking medications for an existing health condition, this might also lead to worse side effects.

How is insomnia diagnosed?

Although you might have all the symptoms, a clear diagnosis may still be necessary, especially if you're not improving even after using the natural tips and methods offered in the book. If this is the case, more intensive techniques may be necessary.

How long before I can see results using natural treatments?

Don't expect an overnight success. Within a week of persistently trying natural sleeping methods, you should be able to notice positive changes in your routine. Keep at it and don't give up until you get quality sleep every night!

What if none of the insomnia treatments work?

Keep in mind that insomnia may be the symptom of another condition. If the problem persists despite all effort, further study may be necessary to find any underlying conditions. Most likely, doctors will have to address the underlying condition for the symptoms – including insomnia – to disappear.

Conclusion

Thank you again for downloading this book!

I hope this book was able to help you to Combat Insomnia and Sleep Problems. Many of these treatments work on different individuals, so it is important to try them all and see what works best for you.

The next step is to keep this book close just in case you know any friends or family that may be suffering from Insomnia and needs to combat their sleep problems. Remember that insomnia is not something you just can fix overnight! The sleep disorder is often caused by week's worth of improper habits so you have to reintroduce new habits to get rid of the problem.

Finally, if you enjoyed this book, please take the time to share your thoughts and post a review on Amazon. It'd be greatly appreciated!

[Click here to leave a review amazon.com](amazon.com)

Thank you!

Jessica Lopez

Join our Mailing List Today to Receive FREE Book Giveaways and Special Offers!

Check Out My Other Books

Below you'll find some of my other popular books that are popular on Amazon and Kindle as well. Simply click on the links below to check them out. Alternatively, you can visit my author page on Amazon to see other work done by me.

[Acne Treatment: How to Treat Acne, Remove Acne, Home Acne, Acne Diets, Acne Control and Acne Medicine](#)

[The Ultimate Guide to Anger Management: How to Control Temper and Conquer Anger](#)

[Weight Loss with Green Juice Diet: Healthy Detox Recipes](#)

[Tea Recipes: Benefits to Help Improve Your Health (Tea Recipes Book 1)](#)

If the links do not work, for whatever reason, you can simply search for these titles on the Amazon website to find them.